Leanne
SPENCER

Cadence

The secret to beating
burnout and performing
in life and work

Leanne

R^ethink

First published in Great Britain in 2022
by Rethink Press (www.rethinkpress.com)

Cover image © Shutterstock | Dreamer Light

Illustrations by Shane Barrell © Leanne Spencer

Contents

	Introduction	1
1	My Story	5
2	Finding Your Cadence	11
	What is the Agile Business Athlete methodology?	11
3	Predict: When Are Your Wimbledons?	15
	Personal events	16
	Professional events	17
	Ask yourself	17
4	Prepare: Sleep	19
	Your bedroom environment	21
	Morning routine	23
	Night-time routine	25
	Ask yourself	27
5	Prepare: Mental Health	29
	Managing your nervous system	30
	Managing neurotransmitters	32
	Using movement	36
	Ask yourself	38

6	**Prepare: Energy**	**41**
	My foundations for fitness	42
	Making time for a mini break	44
	Meeting etiquette	46
	Ask yourself	49
7	**Perform: Respect Your Red Flags**	**51**
	Signs of burnout	53
	Things to watch out for	55
	Ask yourself	57
8	**Recover: Backing Off Beats Burnout**	**59**
	A sliver of recovery	61
	Ways of recovering	62
	Ask yourself	64
	An Example Of An Agile Business Athlete	67
	A Final Message	**73**
	References	**77**
	The Author	**83**

Introduction

I t isn't just that we're doing too much and trying to outperform ourselves in a hyperconnected world; many of us are under-recovered from our efforts and that's when we find ourselves tired, under-energised, lacking resilience and less able to cope with stress. Prioritising recovery through better sleep and managing your mental health are paramount to beat burnout and have more fun.

I wrote this book because I believe burnout will be the next health crisis facing the world. The COVID-19 pandemic has largely made matters worse, with more people reporting poor mental health.[1] According to the UK's Health & Safety Executive, in 2020/21 an estimated 822,000 workers were affected by work-related stress, depression or anxiety.[2] This represents a prevalence rate of 2,480 per 100,000 workers. This rate is not statistically different compared to the previous year. In recent pre-coronavirus pandemic years, the rate of self-reported work-related stress, depression or anxiety had shown signs of increasing. In 2020/21 the rate was higher than the 2018/19 pre-coronavirus levels.

I suffered from burnout in 2012 and, although I made the changes I needed to make before things got to crisis point, I know how devasting it can be. In my current career in wellbeing, I've spoken to many people who say they feel exhausted, have little energy and are depressed. Many are exhibiting classic signs of burnout such as being unable to enjoy things that usually give them pleasure and experiencing mood problems and difficulties sleeping. Life is short and precious, in the most positive sense, so I am making it my mission to show people there is a way to create more balance, beat burnout and have more fun.

The Agile Business Athlete methodology is built around the notion of cadence. Rather than expecting to operate at peak performance all year round, if we introduce cadence, an ebb and flow to the way we manage our energy, then we can perform at our best when we need to. The inspiration comes from athletes, who are generally good at managing and restoring their energy levels by looking ahead to their schedule and identifying the big events; preparing themselves by focusing on their mind, body and wellbeing; performing at a high level when they need to; and then taking a break to allow their minds and bodies to recover. That's the essence of the methodology: Predict, Prepare, Perform and Recover. This book will show you how to apply this methodology to your life.

I'll break down each stage using stories and examples, including tips to help you adopt each principle. I understand you're probably not an actual athlete but a busy professional who doesn't have the time or the professional team that an athlete has around them, and so the suggestions use the concept of the minimal effective dose (MED). This is the smallest change you can make – whether it's to your nutrition, sleep or relaxation practices – that advances your health and wellbeing. Small changes over time can have a surprisingly big effect on how we feel. My goal in writing this book is to motivate you to make a few small changes that feel achievable and, crucially, that you can maintain even in busy times.

Let's get stuck in!

ONE
My Story

It was Friday 23 March 2012, I was working for a market data company based in the City of London and was fifteen years into my career as an account director, a job I had initially loved. I enjoyed the prestige of a city career, the extravagance, the client entertainment and, of course, the salary. In the past few years, however, I'd started to fall out of love with the job and the lifestyle. I couldn't relate to the people around me; I was self-medicating against the stress I felt I was under – my alcohol consumption was increasing and becoming unmanageable. I was making poor food choices, too, and staying out late. Days felt Sisyphean: in Greek mythology, Sisyphus was punished (for cheating death, believe it or not, but that's another story) by being commanded to repeatedly roll a boulder up a hill only to let it roll back down. In other words, every day felt the same. I spent much of my working day checking the clock in the bottom right-hand corner of my screen, wishing days, weeks and months away, rolling from payday to payday. Things had to change, but I seemed to be paralysed at the thought of actually doing anything about it.

Back to that Friday. I was walking to a sales meeting in Monument, on the north side of London Bridge. I felt tired and emotionally drained, but also hopeful because I was expecting a verbal commitment on a sales order. It was a big order and, if I could pull it off, I'd be the hero of the sales team. I walked into the meeting, took off my long woollen coat and sipped my vending machine coffee, taking care not to squeeze the brown plastic cup too hard and cause a spillage. I looked up at my client, and we smiled at each other. Then he hit me with it.

The sales order I was expecting? It wasn't going to happen. His client had pulled out and so there was no need for the data I was hoping to provide.

Rocked by this news, I left the meeting and headed across London Bridge, feeling despondent. I squeezed myself onto the Thameslink train for the short journey home, walked through the front door and sat down to reflect on what had just happened.

I spent the weekend thinking about what to do. After all those months of feeling unable to change my life, this shock jolted me into action. Should I look for another role? Switch careers completely? Do something more drastic? By Sunday evening, I'd made my mind up. I wrote a text to my manager offering my resignation, and by Friday I'd handed back my pass, BlackBerry and laptop and was a free agent. It's not necessarily an approach I'd recommend – I jumped and wondered whether I'd packed a parachute on the way down – but it did work for me.

I took some time out to rest and recover, and then focused on rebuilding my health. I learnt more about sleep in a month than I'd known in my entire life. I began meditating every day, just for five minutes, and really enjoyed that little bit of time to myself. I sold my car and bought a bike, and either cycled or walked everywhere. I started studying other aspects of health, including digestive health, learning about the relationship between our microbiome and mental and physical health. This sparked an interest in food. Before that pivotal day in March, I usually ate ready meals washed down with a bottle or more of red wine, but now I signed up to a vegetable delivery service that worked with spray-free and organic farmers. I frequently had to search online to identify each vegetable and to find ways to cook it. It was, if you like, all celery but not a lot of salary!

To improve my physical fitness, I joined a boxing gym in South London. It's a traditional, under-the-railway-arches boxing gym and quite possibly one of the friendliest in London. I learnt how to box, even having a white-collar boxing match in 2014 (it was a draw, so I'm technically still undefeated). While there, I observed the athletes in the gym, many of them training twice a day, five or six times a week. Despite the rigorous training regime, these athletes didn't appear to burn out. They were able to manage their energy through a combination of good practices such as nutrition, hydration, relaxation, downtime and, most importantly, periods of *recovery*. There was a structure to the way they worked; they didn't expect peak performance all day every day, but rather they'd look ahead to the major events and prepare themselves to be at their best at those times, and schedule in some downtime afterwards. I reflected on the way I'd been living my life, and the way many of us do; there's no rhythm, no cadence to how we do things. We just expect to be 'on' all the time.

I began to consider what I could do to add in more moments of recovery – whether that was a few minutes to daydream while looking out of the window or finishing work to allow myself time in nature each day. I realised two things: first, allowing the mind and body to recover didn't need to take very long. It could be minutes – what I like to call *slivers* of recovery throughout the day. Second, I realised that this was the missing piece for many of us. From here, the Agile Business Athlete methodology began to take shape.

It all begins with cadence.

TWO
Finding Your Cadence

Rather than expecting to operate at peak performance all year round, if we introduce cadence – an ebb and flow to the way we manage our energy – then we can perform at our best when we need to.

What is the Agile Business Athlete methodology?

I often use the example of Serena Williams, one of the most decorated and accomplished athletes of our time. She has won a record number of Grand Slam singles titles. To achieve that, she has beaten Number One players, including her own sister, Venus Williams. She is also one of only two players in the Open Era to have won each major three or more times. Even with this level of success, top athletes won't expect to perform at their best all year round. They will identify the important events in their schedule, and prepare specifically for them, ensuring they're at their peak when these events come around. The preparation will of course involve physical training and practising their own sport, but it will also include managing their nervous system, mental wellbeing, sleep quality and quantity, nutrition and so on.

Of course, top athletes have teams to support and guide them, but looking after these different elements doesn't have to be complicated. We can do it ourselves. How? By focusing on *small things done consistently*. By small things I'm talking about the minimal effective dose (MED), which is the smallest thing you can do that still has a positive effect on your wellbeing. A small (MED) increase in your sleep, mental health and energy can lead to a considerable overall improvement in your health. The key is – it all feels manageable.

Let's get back to the methodology. There are four stages:

Predict: Taking inspiration from those top-performing tennis players, ask yourself 'when are *my* Wimbledons?' When are *the* big events coming up for you? This could be personally or professionally, including any specific goals you have.

Prepare: 'Build your bulletproof' by doubling down on the important elements of good health and wellbeing. We'll spend some time going through these elements, including why they're important and, most importantly, what you can focus on today to make improvements.

Perform: I'm not about to lecture you on how to perform but the key to avoiding burnout is to 'respect your red flags'. The body sends us signs and signals about how it's coping, but we've become adept at ignoring them. Ignore these signs at your peril – that's the way to burnout.

Recover: Backing off beats burnout. During this phase, you allow your mind and body to reset, recover and bring some balance back. I've learnt this the hard way on a few occasions, and I now see recovery as being just as important as the hard work, training and effort – maybe even more important.

In the following chapters, we'll take a deeper dive into each phase. I'll tell stories to bring this to life, and give you tips for each phase that you can apply today with relatively little effort. This stuff is designed to be simple and easy to implement. It doesn't need to be complicated!

THREE

Predict: When Are Your Wimbledons?

One of the biggest tournaments in the tennis calendar is Wimbledon, which will be right up there on any top 100 professional tennis player's priority list. Extending that metaphor, when are your big events coming up? Ask yourself the question, 'when are *my* Wimbledons?' This could be personally or professionally and might include specific goals.

Depending on whether you prefer a long view or a short view of the future, look ahead to the next week, month or quarter. You might even choose to look beyond that to the year ahead, particularly if you know you have a big event coming up, but a short-term view is generally more effective.

Think about both your personal and professional lives.

Personal events

These might include family events, health events or goals you have, such as:

- A child starting school and requiring more support
- You or a member of your family having surgery
- Signing up to a triathlon or marathon
- You or your partner starting a new job
- Moving house
- A new addition to the family – eg a baby or puppy

Professional events

- A quarterly results call
- A promotion or new role within your company
- Launch of a new product line
- Monthly sales targets
- Predicted dip in resources – eg a colleague on annual leave
- Company restructuring

Ask yourself

1. What's coming up in the next one to three months for me?
2. What small tweak could I make to my routine now to prepare?
3. Is everyone who needs to be, aware of these events?

TIP

Mark these events on the calendar and start to enlist the support of friends and family as part of the Prepare stage.

FOUR
Prepare: Sleep

There are a number of theories about why we sleep, and one of the best books on this subject is Professor Matthew Walker's book *Why We Sleep: The new science of sleep and dreams*.[3] Walker says: 'Sleep is the single most effective thing we can do to reset our brain and body health each day – Mother Nature's best effort yet at contra-death.'

Although there is still much we don't know about sleep, here are three great reasons why I personally aim for seven to eight hours every night and advocate others do too.[4]

First, the process of sleeping can help reduce cognitive decline. As we age, we can experience a build-up of plaques in the brain called beta-amyloid plaques, which have been linked to Alzheimer's disease. Studies have shown that sleep helps to flush out these plaques via a process called glymphatic draining. A good night of sleep not only makes you feel better but can also reduce your risk of cognitive decline later in life.

Second, during the phase of sleep called REM (which stands for 'rapid eye movement'), the brain sorts through memories and consolidates learning. It's a vital part of sleep and may partly explain why we tell people to sleep on a problem; sometimes the solution comes to us when we're asleep. I always advise people to 'bed in their learning' with a good night of sleep – for example, after an intense day of workshops or learning.

Last, a good night of sleep helps to regulate the hormones that control or influence our appetites. Ghrelin is responsible for hunger signals and peptide YY is responsible (in part with leptin) for making us feel full. When we have a good night of sleep, those hormones are in balance, and we get signals to eat when appropriate and signals to stop. However, a short night of sleep can unbalance those signals, which can have significant effects on both our energy and weight management, as well as blood sugar control.

Your bedroom environment

View your bedroom as your recovery room. Ideally, it should not contain distractions such as clutter, heavy furniture, piles of clothes or a television. Streamline the room to ensure it's a relaxing and soothing zone in which you can prepare your mind and body for sleep. At night, the optimal condition for sleep is total darkness.

The presence of any light can make it hard to fall asleep and can send confusing messages to the brain about what time of day it is. Our skin has photo receptors on its surface, so if you want to go all-out, attempt to banish all light from the room. I recommend blackout blinds or curtains and an eye mask.

Eliminate any traces of light from LEDs by charging your devices in another room or putting them on flight mode. We don't fully know what the harmful long-term effects are of exposure to so many electromagnetic frequencies (EMFs), but links have been established to insomnia[5] and, according to the World Health Organization's International Agency for Research on Cancer, EMFs are 'possibly carcinogenic to humans.'[6] If you use your phone as an alarm clock, you can still do this with the phone on flight mode. Personally, I don't want to sleep alongside a device that is constantly seeking a Bluetooth and Wi-Fi signal, nor do I want to be tempted to check my phone if I wake up in the night, so I put my phone on flight mode from about 9pm onwards.

Morning routine

In the morning, we want to do the reverse of blocking out the light and be exposed to natural light as soon as we wake. Our circadian rhythms are kick-started by natural light, so as soon as you wake, pull up the blinds or, even better, get outside and fill your retinas with natural light. Move your body gently, by either walking or stretching. Stretching can boost the parasympathetic nervous system and reduce blood pressure,[7] so it's an ideal way to start the day. Exposure to cold water, whether through washing your face or a shower if you can brave it, stimulates the vagus nerve (which is linked to the parasympathetic nervous system), increases alertness and boosts your immune system.[8] It's also crucial to get hourly exposure to natural light, even if only for a few minutes, to maintain

23

a healthy circadian rhythm.[9] If you spend most of your day indoors sitting under harsh, bright light, rarely getting outside, this can negatively impact your ability to sleep well and deeply.

The other type of light to be aware of in relation to sleep is blue light, which, despite its name, doesn't describe the colour but the frequency of light emitted by televisions, smartphones, tablets, laptops and other devices. Blue light suppresses melatonin, which is the hormone that prepares us for sleep,[10] yet many of us sit in front of screens all day and late into the evening. You can wear blue light-blocking glasses, which screen out the blue light. I wear mine from about 7 or 8pm every evening. Many scientific studies have demonstrated the harmful effects of blue light on our ability to sleep, so it's another good reason to put those devices on flight mode or keep them out of the bedroom entirely.

Night-time routine

The evening is when we prepare the body for sleep. The crucial thing is to relax the nervous system. The method I use is called the 'sleep staircase', which you might inadvertently already be following if you have young kids. Typically, a child comes home from school, plays, has tea, perhaps plays some more, then has a bath. After that, they'll put on their pyjamas, have a story and a cuddle in bed, and go to sleep. There may be some variations, but typically that's what we do. This process can be likened to a staircase – descending gradually from busy to calm. At the top is the child coming home from school, and each of the activities is a step on the staircase, with energy levels decreasing with every step, to reach the bed at the bottom.

As adults, we don't tend to do this. Our evening might look like this: arrive home tired and stressed, do a workout, eat a late meal, check emails or flick through our phone, then finish the evening with the 10 o'clock news. We go from the top step to the bottom, missing out the staircase entirely, then wonder why we can't sleep or wake up frequently in the night. We need to look after ourselves like we would our children when it comes to our evening routines and put a staircase in place, each step helping to relax our nervous system and prepare us for sleep.

The last thing to add on the subject of sleep is the sleep window. This is the amount of time you plan to spend in bed relative to the amount of sleep you intend to get. I allow a sleep window of eight to nine hours because I need seven to eight hours' sleep. This allows for the odd wake-up, longer sleep latency than normal (the time it takes to fall asleep) or waking earlier than planned.

Ask yourself

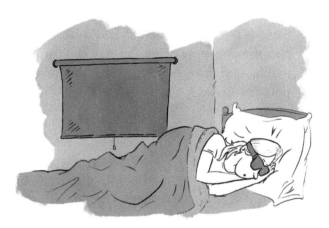

1. What changes could I make to my bedroom to promote restful sleep?

2. What does my sleep staircase look like?

3. Does my sleep window allow for seven to eight hours of quality sleep?

TIP

Sleep is the most democratically available, performance-enhancing strategy you can deploy, and many people underestimate its potency. Could it be your secret weapon?

FIVE

Prepare: Mental Health

What is mental health? According to the World Health Organization, it is the 'state of wellbeing in which the individual realizes his or her own abilities, can cope with the normal stresses of life, can work productively and is able to make a contribution to his or her community.'[11] We all have mental health in the same way we have physical health.

At some point, most of us will experience poor mental health, or know someone who has. As

Pedram Shojai, the Urban Monk, says, 'there's a trillion-dollar healthcare industry that makes money off of chronic diseases that stem from poor lifestyle and uncontrolled stress.'[12]

Managing your nervous system

One of the most effective ways to manage your nervous system is breathwork and meditation. Studies have shown that both these techniques (which can be done separately or at the same time) can reduce blood pressure and resting heart rate and help you control cortisol levels in the body.[13] What I particularly love about these techniques is that they are free and accessible for everyone; they can be done anywhere and at any time.

My favourite breathwork technique is box breathing: imagine the four sides of a box and use that as a guide in your head. It looks like this:

- Inhale for about five seconds while you move up the left side of the box

- Hold the inhalation as you move across the top of the box

- Exhale as you move down the right side of the box

- Hold the exhalation as you move across the bottom of the box

Meditation is another powerful technique I recommend you try. There are many ways to practise, but I favour ten minutes per day first thing in the morning. I don't worry too much about posture or thoughts, but try and relax into it. My partner Antonia does Transcendental Meditation (TM)[14] for twenty minutes twice a day. When I asked her how she makes time for it, she said she sees it as a rest (and her body responds to it as such). It's an interesting way of reframing meditation – would you say no to a ten-minute rest every day?

Many renowned people, including Arianna Huffington,[15] Marc Benioff[16] and Oprah Winfrey,[17] attribute a key part of their success to their TM practice. However, this is something that can work well for everyone.

Managing neurotransmitters

Neurotransmitters play a huge role in mental health, specifically dopamine, oxytocin, serotonin and endorphins – DOSE for short. How can you get your DOSE of happiness? Neurotransmitters are the key.

Dopamine

Dopamine communicates with the reward centre of the brain and plays a role in numerous brain functions including mood, sleep, learning, focus and concentration, motor control and working memory.[18] Here are three ways to manage your dopamine levels:

- Consume more protein: Protein contains amino acids, which are like building blocks for the body.[19]

- Consume probiotics: Excellent sources of probiotics are fermented foods like sauerkraut, kimchi, kombucha or live goat milk kefir.[20]

- Listen to music: Studies have found that listening to music can boost dopamine levels in the brain.[21]

Oxytocin

Oxytocin is a powerful hormone that also acts as a neurotransmitter in the brain. Because of its effect, it's nicknamed the 'bonding and connection hormone' or the 'love hormone'. We experience it when we display generosity or empathy, and when we hug someone.[22] Here are three ways to boost oxytocin:

- Give out hugs: The act of giving someone a hug releases oxytocin, so see how often you can do this in a socially appropriate way.

- Spend time with animals: Studies have shown that spending time with animals (in the case of one study, dogs) releases oxytocin in the body and makes people feel good.[23]

- Give a gift: The act of giving also increases oxytocin and makes us feel good. It could be a random act of kindness, a surprise gift or donating your time to help someone.[24]

Serotonin

Serotonin is another neurotransmitter that impacts every part of your body, from your emotions to your motor skills. It is considered a natural mood stabiliser but is also involved in metabolism and the immune system.[25]

Here are three ways to naturally boost your serotonin levels:

- Eat foods rich in tryptophan and vitamin B6: Chicken, turkey, eggs, cheese, salmon, tuna, spinach, dark leafy greens, chia seeds and nuts are all good sources.[26]

- Sunlight: Ideally the real thing, for about twenty minutes a day, but try to get out in the natural light every hour or so if possible. In winter, you can supplement with vitamin D3 (but test first – you can purchase a test from a direct-to-consumer company or request one from your GP).[27]

- Take a good fish oil: These oils contain high amounts of omega-3 fatty acids called EPA and DHA that are essential for brain health, and boost serotonin.[28]

Endorphins

Endorphins interact with the opiate receptors in the brain to reduce our perception of pain; in this sense, they act similarly to drugs such as morphine and codeine.[29]

Here are three natural ways to boost endorphins:

- Eat chocolate (in moderation): Cocoa
  in dark chocolate increases the level of
  endorphins released into the brain, which
  work to lessen pain and decrease stress.[30]

- Make music: Research has found that
  making music releases endorphins
  that block pain and induce feelings of
  pleasure.[31]

- Try acupuncture: Studies have found that
  acupuncture increases the number of free
  opioid receptors in the brain and triggers
  the release of endorphins.[32]

Using movement

Movement is not only what we as humans were
designed to do, but has several other benefits
related to mental health. Moving our bodies
feels good because it generates endorphins,

which, as we know, make us feel good and increases serotonin in the brain. It also encourages the flow of fresh, oxygenated blood throughout the body, which delivers nutrients to our cells and promotes the creation of new brain cells (neurogenesis).[33]

A study found that just a brisk ten-minute walk a day had the effect of increasing overall mood and energy for up to two hours afterwards, and when done daily for three weeks or more the effects were constant.[34] That's a pretty impressive return on investment.

We've known for a while that movement has a profound effect on mental health, but it doesn't need to be a lot of effort. Walking is very effective, and you can combine it with a commute or a social event like catching up with a friend. In October 2018, it was announced that doctors in Scotland, UK, would start prescribing walks in nature as a treatment for anxiety, high blood pressure and other related conditions.[35] Start moving; it doesn't matter how small those movements are.

Ask yourself

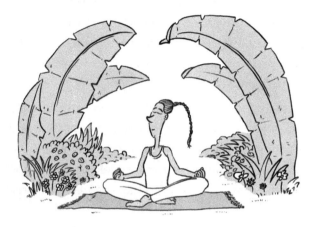

1. What can I do that is meditative?

2. How can I boost my DOSE of happiness?

3. When could I fit a ten-minute brisk walk into my daily routine?

TIP

Think about how you can 'stack' some of these tips into one activity – eg box breathing while on a brisk walk in the natural light. That's a 'three for the effort of one'.

SIX
Prepare: Energy

A few years ago, I learnt a simple lesson about energy (the hard way, of course): it is a limited resource, and we need to be mindful of how we use it. I'd have a hard day or week, then go to the gym and wonder why I couldn't perform to my usual standard. I was frustrated because I hadn't moved all day, so couldn't understand why I didn't have the energy to get active. What I didn't appreciate was that we don't have a separate energy 'jar' for work, the gym and home; it's all drawn from the same bank, whether that's mental, emotional, spiritual or physical energy.

Our energy is a precious and finite resource, and we need to budget it accordingly. The big takeaway for me was deciding how I wanted to spend that energy, and how I would pace myself so that it lasted. If you've used up 50% of your energy working late all week, you should expect less of yourself in the gym or over the weekend, unless you can find ways to replenish it.

It isn't only food and exercise that energise us. People, places and things can warm us up or drain us of our energy. Becoming aware of what those things are for you is powerful.

My foundations for fitness

I have three concepts that are the bedrock of my own fitness – and by 'fitness', I mean fitness for the rigours of daily life or, to put it another way, functional fitness. During one long endurance event, someone asked me what I'd done to prepare for the race. My answer was exactly what you're about to read – so without further ado, here are my *foundations for fitness*:

1. **Steps:** Have a minimum number of steps you take per day. My personal target is 10,000 steps a day, which equates to about 8 km. I have a dog, which makes things easier because she goes out with me every morning. I then make up the steps by keeping active, going on short walks while I take calls and scheduling in tasks throughout the day that require me to move (going to the shops, post office etc).

2. **Standing:** Stand up as a default. Most of us spend our working days sitting down at a desk, which can be bad news for our posture, our spines and our energy levels. I bought a laptop table, which cost me about £35, and I set it up on my desk every morning so I start my day standing

up. I also have a rule that I stand for video calls and when presenting virtually.

3. **Movement snacking:** Here's the killer tip – every hour, do one minute of movement, whether that's five squats, five push-ups, up and down the stairs or anything you can think of that gets your whole body moving. This helps move fresh, oxygenated blood through the body, creates heat and energy and gives you a mini break from your screen. It makes a huge difference.

If you implement these concepts in your everyday life, you'll find that structured exercise is an optional extra on busy days.

Making time for a mini break

A mini break could be as little as a minute, all the way up to thirty minutes. There is no defined time, although there are lots of techniques for taking breaks. Taking short breaks throughout the workday has been proven to increase creativity, productivity, performance and overall wellbeing. I find them essential for managing my energy across a busy day or week.

One study found that taking a break at lunchtime not only increased energy and decreased exhaustion but, if it is done consistently, these benefits got better with time.[36] Here are a few techniques for taking breaks:

- Magic minute: Every hour, take a 1–2-minute break to do a movement snack (energising) or a breathing exercise (relaxing) depending on what you need.
- Schedule in 5-minute breaks between meetings (offer 25-, 55- or 85-minute meeting slots).
- Experiment with Pomodoro® breaks, invented by Francesco Cirillo in the 1980s.[37] The idea is to work for 25 minutes, rest for 5, then work again and so on; on the fourth break, rest for 20–30 minutes.

Most of us will work for several hours before taking a break and that's generally not good for our mind, body and energy levels. Prolonged sitting leads to negative health outcomes and is de-energising. Scheduling in time for mini breaks can be a quick and easy win.

Meeting etiquette

A recent survey found that employees spend on average 15% of their time in meetings.[38] A staggering 55 million meetings are conducted per week, and 67% of employees stated that meetings negatively affected their productivity at work.

If they are run inefficiently and without good meeting etiquette, meetings can suck the energy out of a company's staff. I've put together a few ideas for you to try in your organisation. Whether you run the meeting or not, why not start role-modelling these behaviours?

- If you're the meeting organiser, only invite people who need to be there and send an agenda so they can prepare and bring their best energy to the meeting.

- If you're an attendee, ask questions to establish whether you really do need to be present or could contribute in a different way.

- Does this meeting need to be online or could you switch up the energy and have a phone call instead (which I always consider to be less intense)?

- Any meeting longer than forty-five minutes should include breaks, where attendees can do some movement, get snacks, get a drink, visit the bathrooms or get some natural light.

- In a virtual setting, switch your camera off at strategic times if your energy is low and to give your eyes a rest.

- Try and avoid being static for too long; feel free to encourage others to get up and stretch and even start meetings with an energiser or some gentle movement.

- Pelican rule – if you're the person speaking, then (if you're able to) you stand on one leg and encourage your colleagues to join you. You'd be surprised how quickly people get to the point when they're standing on one leg.

Short, punchy, to-the-point meetings will work wonders for your personal energy and that of your team. By adopting some of the best practices listed above, you'll boost the creativity, productivity and performance of yourself and your teams.

Ask yourself

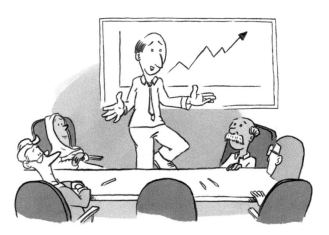

1. What movement snacks can I introduce every hour?

2. How can I contribute to better meetings in my company?

3. How can I build mini breaks into my working day?

TIP

Magic minute: What could you do for one minute every hour that either energises you (movement snack) or relaxes you (breathwork)?

SEVEN

Perform: Respect Your Red Flags

A few years ago, I woke up on a Monday morning feeling terrible. I felt as though an invisible force was pushing me down on the bed, pinning me to the mattress. When I tried to open my eyes, I had an aversion to light and could only squint or close my eyes again. My mouth was dry, I felt nauseous and was incredibly lethargic. Eventually, driven by the need to go to the loo, I peeled myself off the mattress and shuffled downstairs on my bum, and into the bathroom. I had to climb back up the stairs on my hands and knees and get back into bed, where I stayed almost solidly for three days. At the end of day three I felt slightly better, so went for a short walk in my local park. I soon realised my energy was nowhere near recovered – I had to stop at the benches every 100 metres or so and sit down for a few minutes. It was several days before I felt close to my normal self. My partner and I called this strange illness the 'mystery sickness'. It came back again after three months and again three months after that.

In hindsight, there was no mystery at all. I was simply doing too much and not respecting my red flags. These flags are indicators that you may be pushing a bit too hard and heading for burnout. I was working long and varied hours, studying and writing a book in my spare time and doing double time down at the gym. I had ignored the signs (anhedonia: an inability to take pleasure from activities you usually enjoy;

mild insomnia; and libido and appetite issues) and my body intervened by manifesting physical illness. As a result, I slowed down, built in more recovery (see the next chapter) and adjusted my pace of life. I'm pleased to say I haven't experienced the mystery sickness since.

Back to you. You've identified the big events coming up for you and you've concentrated on sleep, mental health and energy to ensure you can perform at your best. Now you've reached the Perform stage and need to be aware of what your red flags are.

Signs of burnout

The indicators vary from person to person and depending on the situation you're in but being aware of them will help you stay healthy and perform optimally. Two psychologists, Herbert Freudenberger and Gail North, created the twelve stages of burnout, a helpful guide that walks you through the spectrum of mild stress to burnout.[39] My company Bodyshot Performance has adapted the guide with some tips on what to do if this is you or someone you know.[40]

Here are the twelve stages, as defined by Freudenberger and North:

- Compulsion to prove oneself
- Working harder
- Neglecting needs
- Displacement of conflicts
- Revision of values
- Denial of emerging problems
- Withdrawal
- Odd behavioural changes
- Depersonalisation
- Inner emptiness
- Depression
- Burnout syndrome

Chronic stress and burnout can manifest in different ways but check out our guide if you recognise any of these stages and do take action.

Things to watch out for

Examples of red flags are listed below; you may find the acronym REDFLAGS helps you remember them. You might only experience some of these, or each of them at different times:

- R: rage, or quick to become angry
- E: emptiness
- D: despondency or depression
- F: fatigue
- L: low mood
- A: anhedonia (loss of pleasure in activities you normally enjoy)
- G: guilt or a feeling of letting people down
- S: self-doubt or low self-esteem

This isn't a comprehensive list and of course there are physical symptoms, too, such as headaches, unexplained aches and pains and frequent illness such as common colds, but it gives you clues about what to look out for.

It's important to note that if you are experiencing any of these symptoms in a way that feels different or more persistent, seek the advice of your doctor or speak to a professional.

Ask yourself

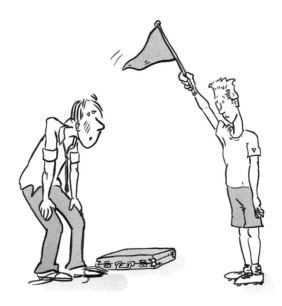

1. What are *my* red flags?

2. Do I schedule time to check in with myself on how I'm feeling?

3. What's the one thing I can do straight away if I see one of these flags go up?

TIP

Identify that one thing that you would
do if a red flag goes up and have a visual
reminder somewhere in your office or home
environment.

EIGHT

Recover: Backing Off Beats Burnout

In March 2012, my partner Antonia and I set off on our biggest challenge to date, the Arctic Circle Race (ACR). The ACR is a 160 km cross-country ski race in Greenland and is billed as the world's toughest ski race. It's a three-day event and you overnight in two-person tents erected for you in camp. It's gruelling and requires extreme levels of fitness and considerable mental fortitude. We signed up because Antonia's father was profoundly ill with Alzheimer's disease and we wanted to raise £10,000 for the Alzheimer's Research charity (spoiler alert: we did!). We trained for a week in Austria and did lots of roller-skiing in Richmond and Dulwich Parks in South London, and we both have good levels of fitness, but nothing prepared us for what we experienced within just an hour of setting off.

We subsequently discovered the elevation on day one alone was the equivalent of climbing Snowdon two and a half times – had we known that, we'd have climbed more mountains in training. The weather had obliterated the tracks so we couldn't ski in the conventional way. Within minutes, we'd fallen to the back of the pack and couldn't see the other athletes, and what I thought I'd love about the experience – the mountains, the solitude and the rawness of nature – I actually found intimidating and overwhelming. I had meltdown after meltdown and experienced anxiety for the first time. I told Antonia in no uncertain terms that I was going

to quit as soon as we got into camp at the end
of the day – if we made it that far.

A sliver of recovery

After over twelve hours of skiing across 55 km
of rugged terrain, the camp was finally in sight.
I still had every intention of quitting. As we
skied closer, I saw one of the volunteers, a local
Inuit woman wearing a thick fur-lined coat,
looking out towards me with her arms open. I
got within a few metres of her and realised the
offer of a hug was for me. I skied into her arms,
and we held each other in a tight embrace for
what seemed like minutes but was probably
only about sixty seconds. I began to withdraw,
thinking I ought to let this woman go, but as I
did so she pulled me back in again. When we
did separate, Antonia was able to persuade me
to go the changing tent and put on fresh clothes,
and then to the food tent and finally to our tent

for the night. I didn't quit, and two days later we skied across the finish line together.

Had I not had that hug, though – that sixty-second *sliver* of recovery – I don't think I would have gone on. In that minute, I was able to get some headspace, back off and recalibrate. That moment was pivotal to my being able to finish the race.

Ways of recovering

Your version of this *sliver* of recovery probably won't involve an Inuit woman, or possibly even a hug (although it might), but there will be something you can do on an hourly basis that creates that headspace for you.

The suggestions in the mental health chapter also apply to recovery. Here are five more ideas you could try – remember consistency is key:

- Magic minute of breathing: Set a timer for sixty seconds, close your eyes and breathe deeply.

- Daydream: Head for the nearest window and let your eyes and mind wander.

- Natural light: Enjoy the benefit of fresh air and the serotonin we get from the sun.

- Eye contact: If you have a dog, try staring into their eyes and get a big dose of oxytocin.

- Converse: Enjoy a moment of connection with another human being, ideally in person.

Ask yourself

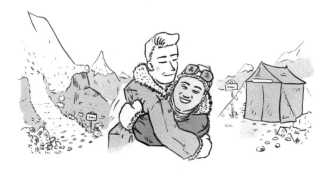

1. What slivers of recovery can I incorporate into my day?

2. What makes me feel lighter or more relaxed? Create a shortlist.

3. What one thing can I implement today?

TIP

Take five minutes for yourself every hour
by offering 25- or 55-minute meeting slots;
that's your chance to take refreshment
breaks between meetings and schedule in
those slivers of recovery.

An Example Of An Agile Business Athlete

Alex is the marketing director of a large multi-national firm based in London. She's in her early forties, married and has two young children with her partner. She commutes to work most days, a journey of over forty minutes. She typically passes the time checking emails or making notes. Alex likes running, fitness and walking and enjoys being active with her family, exploring local sights and countryside.

Alex uses the Agile Business Athlete methodology to help her achieve her health goals, which are broadly to have good energy for her young family and to maintain good health as she enters old age (longevity of healthspan).

Here's how Alex applies the methodology in practice:

Predict: The big upcoming event for Alex in her personal life is her youngest child starting school (a big deal for all the family). In her professional life, Alex is heavily involved in a new acquisition that her company is making. Both these events are going to require her best energy, focus and efficiency.

Prepare: Alex prepares for these upcoming events by making a few changes to her lifestyle. She goes to bed thirty minutes earlier every night to get that extra sleep, which she finds makes a big difference to her mood and energy. As a family, they reduce the number of social events they go to, so they don't feel like they're rushing around so much at weekends. Lastly, Alex will get in a few extra runs and exercise minutes leading up to these big events, because she knows she will almost certainly have less time for the next few weeks.

Perform: While she's going through the busier part of her life, Alex will work hard but avoid overdoing it by sticking to her daily nonnegotiables. Crucially, she'll watch out for her red flags, and perhaps ask her partner to look out for them too. Alex has identified that these are low/irritable mood, difficulties sleeping and suppressed appetite. If she spots these things creeping in, she knows she needs to put the brakes on a bit.

Recover: Once the acquisition is complete and her child is settled at school, Alex can relax a little and take a couple of days off to do something fun and restorative. The family will arrange a few social events and perhaps make plans for a summer holiday or an adventure during half-term. Alex will take a lunch hour again and start exercising more.

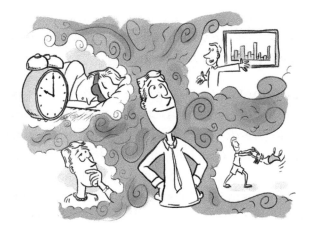

And that's how it works. Alex uses the cadence of the Agile Business Athlete methodology to manage her life so that although there are busy and challenging times, she's able to avoid burning out. She focuses on small changes that have a big impact, and always looks ahead to identify when the demanding times will be.

Of course, the unexpected will sometimes happen in our personal and professional lives, but if you follow the advice in this book about sleep, mental health and energy, you'll feel more resilient and be well on your way to dealing with the surprises.

A Final Message

My goal has been to keep this book simple, use stories where possible to demonstrate the principles and give you some strategies that you can adopt to help create the cadence to cope with a busy life. I understand you have many things to think about, and I have no doubt time is in short supply. If you're unsure where to start, then just pick one thing that feels easy to do.

Small, consistent changes have a powerful effect over time. The ideas in this book do not have to take a lot of time. Sir Dave Brailsford, who guided the Sky Cycling Team among others, used the term 'the aggregation of marginal gains' to describe one of his principles for success and it can definitely be applied to health and wellbeing.[41] If you can introduce a few small changes to a few areas of your life, you'll enjoy significant benefits.

I recall a conversation I had several years ago with a woman who had had a successful business career and was at that time chair of a start-up. She was frustrated because she felt she had no time between meetings to collect her thoughts and decompress before the next meeting began. She had tried meditation using various apps but didn't feel she was getting any benefit from it. I was struck by previous conversations where she'd told me about her hobbies and I suggested that perhaps she found these things meditative, and she agreed. She came up with an idea that was to change everything: she brought one of her smaller craft projects with her and spent a few minutes between meetings working on that, and she felt much more composed going into the next meeting. This is a perfect example of what slivers of recovery, mere minutes in a day, can do for your mood and energy, and how they can turn you from a stressed-out, busy professional into a happy, healthy and resilient Agile Business Athlete.

I wish you all the best.

References

1   Office for Health Improvement & Disparities,
    Coronavirus (COVID-19), 'Covid-19: mental health and
    wellbeing surveillance report', (updated 18 November
    2021), www.gov.uk/government/publications/covid
    -19-mental-health-and-wellbeing-surveillance-report
    /2-important-findings-so-far, accessed 14 February 2022
2   Health and Safety Executive (HSE), 'Work-related stress,
    depression or anxiety statistics in Great Britain, 2021',
    (16 December 2021), www.hse.gov.uk/statistics/causdis
    /stress.pdf, accessed 14 February 2022
3   M Walker, *Why We Sleep: The new science of sleep and
    dreams* (Penguin, 2018)
4   M Walker, *Why We Sleep: The new science of sleep and
    dreams* (Penguin, 2018)
5   T Barsam, M R Monazzam, A A Haghdoost et al, 'Effect
    of extremely low frequency electromagnetic field expo-
    sure on sleep quality in high voltage substations', *Iranian
    Journal of Environmental Health Science & Engineering*, 9(15)
    (2012), https://doi.org/10.1186/1735-2746-9-15
6   World Health Organization, 'Electromagnetic fields and
    public health: mobile phones', (Fact sheet, 8 October

2014), www.who.int/news-room/fact-sheets/detail /electromagnetic-fields-and-public-health-mobile-phones, accessed 4 February 2022

7   J Ko, D Deprez, K Shaw et al, 'Stretching is superior to brisk walking for reducing blood pressure in people with high-normal blood pressure or stage I hypertension', *Journal of Physical Activity and Health*, 18(1) (2021), 21–28, https://journals.humankinetics.com/view/journals/jpah /18/1/article-p21.xml, accessed 14 March 2022

8   R Nall, 'Are there any health benefits to a cold shower?', *Medical News Today* (12 July 2019), www .medicalnewstoday.com/articles/325725, accessed 14 February 2022

9   C Blume, C Garbazza and M Spitschan, 'Effects of light on human circadian rhythms, sleep and mood', *Somnologie*, 23 (2019), 147–156, https://doi.org/10.1007 /s11818-019-00215-x

10   Harvard Medical School, 'Blue light has a dark side: What is blue light? The effect blue light has on your sleep and more', *Harvard Health Publishing* (7 July 2020), www.health.harvard.edu/staying-healthy/blue-light-has -a-dark-side, accessed 14 February 2022

11   World Health Organization (WHO), 'Mental health: strengthening our response', (Fact sheet, 30 March 2018), www.who.int/news-room/fact-sheets/detail/mental -health-strengthening-our-response, accessed 14 February 2022

12   P Shojai, *The Urban Monk: Eastern wisdom and modern hacks to stop time and find success, happiness, and peace* (Rodale Press Inc, 2016)

13   D H Craighead, T C Heinbockel, K A Freeberg et al, 'Time-efficient inspiratory muscle strength training lowers blood pressure and improves endothelial function, NO bioavailability, and oxidative stress in midlife/older adults with above-normal blood pressure', *Journal of the American Heart Association*, 10(3) (2021), https://doi

.org/10.1161/JAHA.121.020980; A Zaccaro, A Piarulli, M
Laurino et al, 'How breath-control can change your life:
A systematic view on psycho-physiological correlates of
slow breathing', *Frontiers in Human Neuroscience*, 12(353)
(2018), https://doi.org/10.3389/fnhum.2018.00353; X Ma,
Z-Q Yue, A-Q Gong et al, 'The effect of diaphragmatic
breathing on attention, negative affect and stress in
healthy adults', *Frontiers in Psychology*, 8(874) (2017),
https://doi.org/10.3389/fpsyg.2017.00874

14   Transcendental Meditation, https://uk.tm.org, accessed 4
February 2022

15   Transcendental Meditation, https://uk.tm.org/web
/learn-tm/arianna-huffington, accessed 4 February
2022; Transcendental Meditation, *'The Huffington Post*
editors learn to counter work stress with meditation', (15
May 2015), https://tmhome.com/news-events/arianna
-huffington-post-meditation, accessed 14 February 2022

16   J Lockhart and M Hicken, '14 Executives who swear by
meditation', *Insider* (9 May 2012), www.businessinsider
.com/ceos-who-meditate-2012-5?r=US&IR=T#hedge-fund
-manager-ray-dalio-uses-transcendental-meditation-to
-check-his-ego-1, accessed 14 February 2022

17   O Winfrey, 'What Oprah knows for sure about finding
the fullest expression of yourself', *The Oprah Magazine*
(February 2021), www.oprah.com/health/oprah-on
-stillness-and-meditation-oprah-visits-fairfield-iowa,
accessed 4 February 2022

18   S Watson, 'Dopamine: The pathway to pleasure', *Harvard
Health Publishing* (20 July 2021), www.health.harvard.edu
/mind-and-mood/dopamine-the-pathway-to-pleasure,
accessed 4 February 2022

19   K Peuhkuri, N Sihvola and R Korpela, 'Dietary proteins
and food-related reward signals', *Food & Nutrition
Research*, 55 (2011), doi: 10.3402/fnr.v55i0.5955

20   K Berkheiser, '12 dopamine supplements to
boost your mood', *Healthline* (1 August 2018),

www.healthline.com/nutrition/dopamine-supplements#:, accessed 15 February 2022

21 S McGilchrist, 'Music "releases mood-enhancing chemical in the brain"', BBC News (9 January 2011), www.bbc.co.uk/news/health-12135590, accessed 14 February 2022

22 S Watson, 'Oxytocin: The love hormone', *Harvard Health Publishing* (20 July 2021), www.health.harvard.edu/mind-and-mood/oxytocin-the-love-hormone, accessed 4 February 2022

23 A Beetz, K Uvnäs-Moberg, H Julius et al, 'Psychosocial and psychophysiological effects of human-animal interactions: the possible role of oxytocin', *Frontiers in Psychology*, 3(234) (2012), www.frontiersin.org/articles/10.3389/fpsyg.2012.00234/full, accessed 14 March 2022

24 Cedars-Sinai Staff, 'The science of kindness', Cedars-Sinai Blog (13 February 2019), www.cedars-sinai.org/blog/science-of-kindness.html, accessed 15 March 2022

25 S Watson, 'Seratonin: The natural mood booster', *Harvard Health Publishing* (20 July 2021), www.health.harvard.edu/mind-and-mood/serotonin-the-natural-mood-booster, accessed 4 February 2022

26 T A Jenkins, J C Nguyen, K E Polglaze et al, 'Influence of tryptophan and serotonin on mood and cognition with a possible role of the gut-brain axis', *Nutrients*, 8(1) (2016), 56, https://doi.org/10.3390/nu8010056

27 R Nall, 'What are the benefits of sunlight: Sunlight and serotonin', *Healthline* (1 April 2019), www.healthline.com/health/depression/benefits-sunlight#, accessed 15 February 2022

28 UCSF Benioff Children's Hospital Oakland, 'Omega-3 fatty acids, vitamin D may control brain serotonin, affecting behavior and psychiatric disorders', *ScienceDaily* (25 February 2015), www.sciencedaily.com/releases/2015/02/150225094109.htm, accessed 14 February 2022

29 Harvard Medical School, 'Endorphins: The brain's natural pain reliever', *Harvard Health Publishing* (20 July 2021),

www.health.harvard.edu/mind-and-mood/endorphins
-the-brains-natural-pain-reliever, accessed 4 February
2022

30 A Nehlig, 'The neuroprotective effects of cocoa flavanol
and its influence on cognitive performance', *British
Journal of Clinical Pharmacology*, 75(3) (2013), 716–727,
https://doi.org/10.1111/j.1365-2125.2012.04378.x

31 R I Dunbar, K Kaskatis, I MacDonald et al, 'Performance
of music elevates pain threshold and positive affect:
implications for the evolutionary function of music',
Evolutionary Psychology, 10(4) (2012), 688–702, https://
pubmed.ncbi.nlm.nih.gov/23089077, accessed 14
February 2022

32 J S Han, 'Acupuncture and endorphins', *Neuroscience
Letters*, 361(1–3), 258–61, https://pubmed.ncbi.nlm.nih.gov
/15135942, accessed 4 February 2022

33 A Yeager, 'How exercise reprograms the brain', *The
Scientist* (1 November 2018), www.the-scientist.com
/features/this-is-your-brain-on-exercise-64934
15 Feburary 2022

34 M K Edwards and P D Loprinzi, 'Experimental effects of
brief, single bouts of walking and meditation on mood
profile in young adults', *Health Promotion Perspectives*, 8(3)
(2018), 171–178, https://hpp.tbzmed.ac.ir/Article/hpp-
20320, accessed 15 February 2022

35 P Dockrill, 'Doctors in Scotland are literally prescribing
nature to their patients', *ScienceAlert* (9 October 2018),
www.sciencealert.com/doctors-in-scotland-are-literally
-prescribing-nature-to-patients-shetland-gps-pilot
-benefits-health-mental, accessed 15 February 2022

36 A Kohll, 'New study shows correlation between
employee engagement and the long-lost lunch break',
Forbes (29 May 2018), www.forbes.com/sites/alankohll
/2018/05/29/new-study-shows-correlation-between
-employee-engagement-and-the-long-lost-lunch-break,
accessed 15 February 2022

37 F Cirillo, 'The Pomodoro® Technique', Not Harder, https://francescocirillo.com/pages/pomodoro-technique, accessed 4 February 2022

38 C Chen, 'Shocking meeting statistics in 2021 that will take you by surprise', otter.ai Blog (24 December 2020), https://blog.otter.ai/meeting-statistics/#, accessed 15 February 2022

39 H J Freudenberger and G North, *Women's Burnout: How to spot it, how to reverse it and how to prevent it* (Penguin Books, 1986)

40 You can access the guide at www.bodyshotperformance .com/resources/the-12-stages-of-burnout or by typing '12 stages of burnout Bodyshot' into a web browser

41 Richard Moore, *Mastermind: How Dave Brailsford reinvented the wheel* (BackPage Press, 2013)

The Author

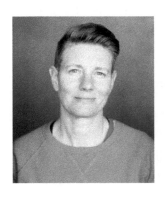

Leanne Spencer is a keynote speaker and wellbeing consultant. Leanne began her career in sales and spent over fifteen years working in the City of London before leaving in 2012 to set up her own business, Bodyshot Performance Limited, after suffering from burnout. Bodyshot specialises in creating happy, healthy and resilient teams, working with companies such as iTech Media, DAZN, Britvic and Zurich Insurance.

Cadence is Leanne's third book, after the bestselling books *Rise and Shine* and *Remove the Guesswork*. She lives in South London but escapes to the countryside whenever possible. Leanne loves sport, fitness, reading, hiking, business, podcasting and spending time with her wife, rescue cat Puss, and Kami the Romanian rescue dog. Leanne is also a Bear Grylls Survival Instructor.

You can follow Leanne on social media or visit her website for videos and blogs:

🌐 www.leannespencer.co.uk
❦ www.facebook.com/leannespencerkeynote
in www.linkedin.com/in/leannespencer1975
◉ @leannespencerkeynote